what you should know

Congestive Heart Failure

BETTERWAY BOOKS

what you should know

Congestive Heart Failure

Written by Douglas Wetherill, MS,
and Dean J. Kereiakes, MD, FACC
Illustrated by Laura L. Seeley

To:

Jenna, David, Andrew, Nicky,

and

Anne — who holds it all together.

— Dean

We must also acknowledge the generous support of the following individuals: Angela Ginty, Peggy Marquette, Janette Weisbrodt, Lynne Haag, Dorothy and Steven Stoller, Cathy Walker, Paul Neff, Karen Perl, Janice Caputo, Richard Hunt, Phil Sexton, and Sara Dumford.

We would also like to extend our appreciation to The McGraw-Hill Companies for permission to use their adapted illustrations.

Treatment Disclaimer

This book is for education purposes, not for use in the treatment of medical conditions. It is based on skilled medical opinion as of the date of publication. However, medical science advances and changes rapidly. Furthermore, diagnosis and treatment are often complex and involve more than one disease process or medical issue to determine proper care. If you believe you may have a medical condition described in the book, consult your doctor.

Table of Contents

Introduction

Congestive heart failure (CHF). This term probably does not roll off the tip of your tongue. Yet CHF is the fastest growing form of cardiovascular disease in the United States. It has been estimated that 2% of the U.S. population over 40 years old has CHF, and CHF is the most frequent diagnosis in the growing geriatric patient population.

This book defines CHF. It reviews some of the risk factors for CHF and explores possible treatment options. Please remember cardiovascular disease may be genetic or inherited. Also, it is important that you discuss **your** specific medical condition with **your** doctor.

It may be easier for you to understand CHF and how it develops once you understand how the heart works. Follow along — we'll start slowly.

Heart Anatomy

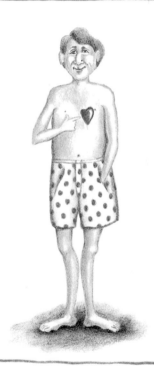

The heart

The heart is a muscle.
It pumps blood to the
head and the body.
It is about the size
of your fist and sits
just to the left of the
middle of your chest.

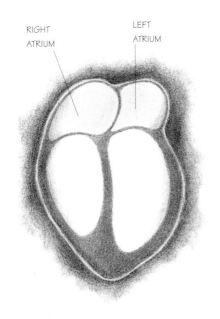

RIGHT
ATRIUM

LEFT
ATRIUM

The heart is asymmetrical. It is made up of 4 chambers. The top 2 chambers are called the **atria**. The atria collect blood returning to the heart. The atria then dump the blood into the ventricles.

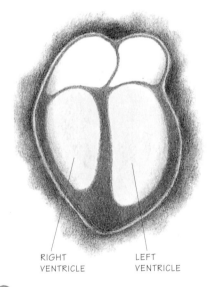

RIGHT
VENTRICLE

LEFT
VENTRICLE

The bottom 2 chambers are called the **ventricles**. The ventricles are larger than the atria, and the left one is more muscular. When the ventricles contract, they force blood out of the heart to different parts of the body.

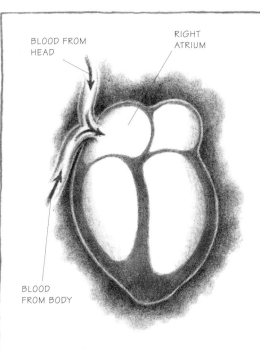

BLOOD FROM HEAD

RIGHT ATRIUM

BLOOD FROM BODY

The body uses food and oxygen carried by the blood. The blood returning to the heart has had oxygen removed. This "deoxygenated" blood collects in the **right atrium**.

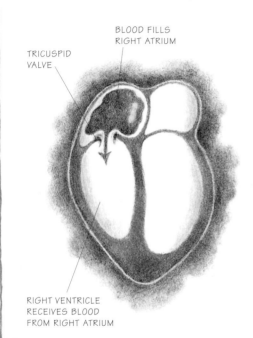

TRICUSPID
VALVE

BLOOD FILLS
RIGHT ATRIUM

RIGHT VENTRICLE
RECEIVES BLOOD
FROM RIGHT ATRIUM

The blood in the **right atrium** is forced through the **tricuspid valve** (one-way valve) and goes into the **right ventricle**.

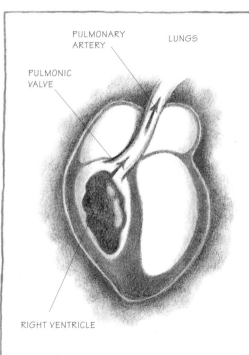

PULMONARY ARTERY

LUNGS

PULMONIC VALVE

RIGHT VENTRICLE

The **tricuspid valve** closes. The **right ventricle** contracts and pumps blood through the **pulmonic valve**. The blood travels through the **pulmonary artery** to the **lungs** where it picks up oxygen.

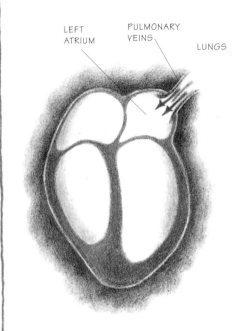

LEFT ATRIUM

PULMONARY VEINS

LUNGS

Once the blood picks up oxygen in the lungs, it returns to the heart through the **pulmonary veins** and collects inside the **left atrium**. The oxygen-rich blood is ready to be used by the body again.

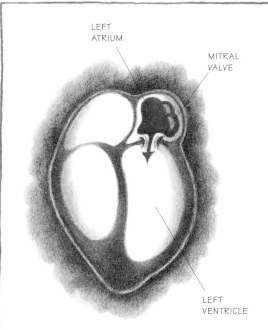

LEFT
ATRIUM

MITRAL
VALVE

LEFT
VENTRICLE

The **left atrium** contracts and sends the blood through the **mitral valve** (another one-way valve) and into the **left ventricle**.

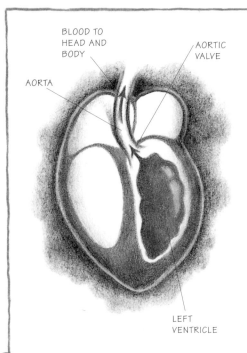

BLOOD TO
HEAD AND
BODY

AORTIC
VALVE

AORTA

LEFT
VENTRICLE

The **mitral valve** closes. The **left ventricle** contracts and pumps oxygenated blood through the **aortic valve** into the **aorta**. The blood then travels through the **aorta**, providing life-sustaining oxygen and nutrients to the body.

So:

1) Blood with lower oxygen content collects in the right atrium.

2) The right ventricle pumps blood to the lungs.

3) Oxygen-rich blood collects in the left atrium.

4) The left ventricle pumps oxygen-rich blood to the head and the rest of the body. The amount of blood that is pumped out of the left ventricle is called the **ejection fraction**. The ejection fraction is indicative of how well the heart is working.

Ejection fraction

A little more than half of the blood in the left ventricle is pumped out of the heart with each beat. The amount of blood that is pumped out is called the **ejection fraction**. A **normal** ejection fraction is 55% or greater.

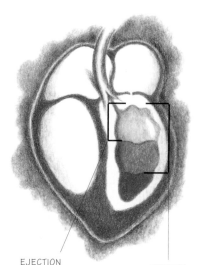

EJECTION FRACTION FOR SOMEONE WITH CONGESTIVE HEART FAILURE

NORMAL EJECTION FRACTION

Congestive heart failure (CHF) occurs when the left ventricle has been weakened and the heart does not properly pump the blood. Someone with congestive heart failure may have an ejection fraction of **less than 40%**, and sometimes even **less than 20%**. Instead of pumping 2 to 3 ounces of blood with each beat, someone with CHF may only pump 1 to 2 ounces of blood with each beat.

Thus, the "F" in CHF means **failure** of the heart to pump blood adequately. The force with which the blood is pumped is reduced, and the quantity of blood pumped with each beat (**ejection fraction**) may fall. The **ejection fraction** of the **left ventricle** is usually determined by 1 of 3 tests:

1) an **echo**
2) a **catheterization** or
3) a MUGA

1. Echo

A sound-wave probe is held against the outside of the chest. The probe uses a Doppler image (similar to a sonogram) to show how effectively the heart muscle is pumping and to measure blood flow.

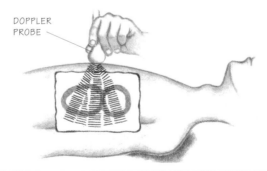

DOPPLER PROBE

2. Catheterization

A small incision is made in the leg or arm artery. A thin tube called a catheter is inserted into either the leg or arm artery and pushed up into the heart. Angiographic contrast, or "dye," is injected through the catheter into the left ventricle so that the function of the left ventricle can be observed directly.

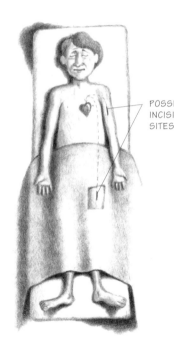

POSSIBLE INCISION SITES

3. Radionuclide ventriculogram (MUGA)

Nuclear dye is injected into the blood. X-ray pictures are taken to determine how much dye is being pumped out of the heart during each beat. This test does not require a catheter to be inserted into the heart.

What are the symptoms of congestive heart failure?

1) Shortness of breath, noted at first during physical exertion. If the disease progresses, shortness of breath may occur even when resting.
2) Physical activity limitations (fatigue)
3) Waking from sleep due to shortness of breath
4) Swelling in the legs and feet and weight gain due to fluid "buildup" or retention (sometimes called **edema**)

How does CHF impact other areas of the body?

Imagine for a moment that you are sitting in rush-hour traffic. Everyone is trying to use the same road at the same time. There just is not enough room to handle all the cars. So, what happens? Traffic becomes backed up.

That is very similar to what happens in the body with congestive heart failure.

Because less blood is pumped out of the damaged heart, the heart cannot keep up with all the blood returning to the heart. Blood backs up in the heart and the rest of the body, causing a buildup of fluid in the tissues.

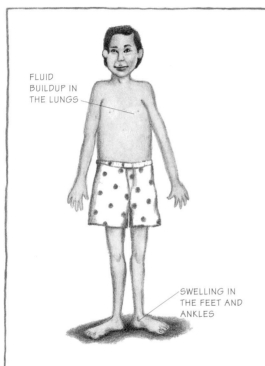

FLUID BUILDUP IN THE LUNGS

SWELLING IN THE FEET AND ANKLES

Fluid congestion in the tissues (**edema**) usually results in swelling of the legs and ankles. Fluid may also build up in the lungs. Fluid buildup in the lungs results in difficulty breathing, especially when lying down.

You may be surprised to learn that the decreased ability of the heart to contract also affects the kidneys' function. The kidneys act like a water filter for your blood. Blood flows through the kidneys so that impurities can be removed.

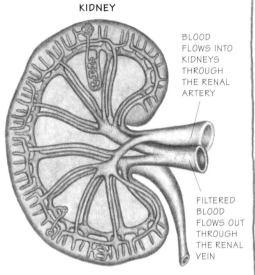

BLOOD FLOWS INTO KIDNEYS THROUGH THE RENAL ARTERY

FILTERED BLOOD FLOWS OUT THROUGH THE RENAL VEIN

PERMISSION GRANTED BY THE McGRAW-HILL COMPANIES FOR USE OF ADAPTED ILLUSTRATION BY H. McMURTRIE and J. RIKEL, *THE COLORING REVIEW GUIDE TO HUMAN ANATOMY*, 1991, Wm. C. BROWN PUBLISHERS.

The amount of blood received by the kidneys varies in direct proportion to the amount of blood pumped by the heart. When the heart pumps less blood, the kidneys feel "starved" and retain sodium (found in salt) and water, resulting in fluid retention.

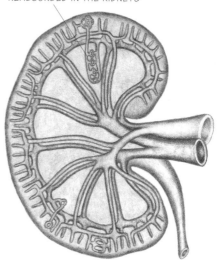

SALT AND WATER ARE REABSORBED IN THE KIDNEYS

PERMISSION GRANTED BY THE McGRAW-HILL COMPANIES FOR USE OF ADAPTED ILLUSTRATION BY H. McMURTRIE and J. RIKEL, *THE COLORING REVIEW GUIDE TO HUMAN ANATOMY*, 1991, Wm. C. BROWN PUBLISHERS.

Here's a quick summary.

1) The fractional amount of blood pumped out of the **left ventricle** is called the **ejection fraction**. For a normal individual, the ejection fraction is about 55%. Someone with congestive heart failure usually has an ejection fraction of less than 40%.

2) When the left ventricle does not pump properly, fluid may build up in the lungs (causing difficulty breathing) and in the body (causing swelling or **edema**).

How does the left ventricle become damaged?

Like all muscles, the heart needs oxygen to work properly. The arteries that supply oxygen-rich blood to the heart are called **coronary arteries**. Damage to the heart muscle occurs when these arteries become blocked and cannot supply enough blood to the working heart muscle.

Arteries and Coronary Arteries

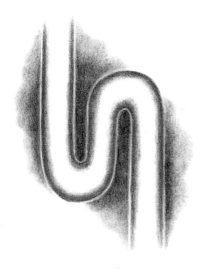

Arteries carry blood much the same way a plumbing system carries water throughout a house.

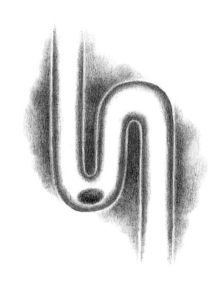

Over time, debris traveling through the pipes may collect in a bend. Debris that collects and restricts water flow is known as a clog or a blockage.

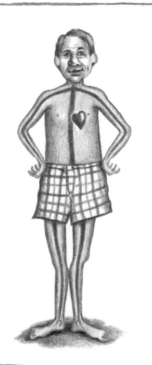

Arteries and veins
wind throughout the
body carrying blood.
Arteries carry blood
away from the heart.
Veins carry blood back
to the heart.

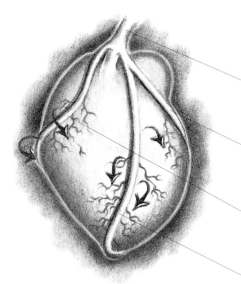

The heart has its own arteries to provide blood to the heart muscle.

The **aorta** supplies blood to the arteries of the heart as well as to the rest of the body.

The **circumflex artery** supplies blood to the lateral or side aspect of the heart.

The **right coronary artery** provides blood to the back or underside of the heart.

The **left anterior descending artery** supplies blood to the front of the heart.

31

To give you some idea of their size, the **coronary arteries** are only about the size of a strand of spaghetti.

(APPROXIMATE SIZE OF SPAGHETTI)

At birth, the inside of the arteries, including the coronary arteries, is slippery — similar to a nonstick pan. The blood cells (represented by the small cars) flow smoothly through the arteries.

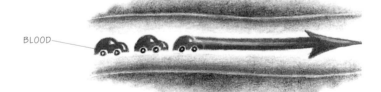

BLOOD

What happens to an artery
during a person's lifetime?

Fatty streaks in the arteries start to develop in the first decade of life as a result of lipids moving into the cell wall of the artery.

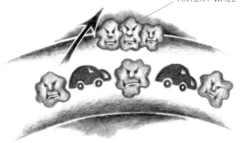

LIPIDS MOVING INTO THE ARTERY WALL

These fatty streaks may become more advanced **atherosclerotic lesions** in the presence of risk factors such as smoking, high blood pressure, obesity, high cholesterol, and physical inactivity. The fatty streaks may then progress to **atheromas** and **fibroatheromas**, which are more "advanced lesions" and are often referred to as **plaque.**

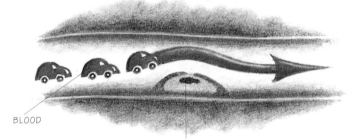

BLOOD

ATHEROSCLEROTIC LESION

Buildups may occur in more than one place in the artery. They may occur at different points along the length of the artery.

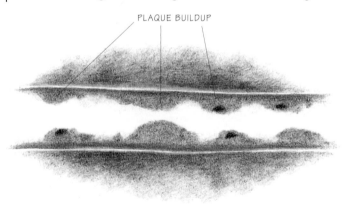

PLAQUE BUILDUP

The total closure of the artery may occur due to: a) the **buildup** of plaque, b) the formation of a blood clot on the plaque, c) the plaque **rupturing** and causing a larger blood clot to form, or d) the plaque rupturing off the artery wall and lodging in a narrowed section of the artery. The complete blockage of the artery is called an **occlusion**.

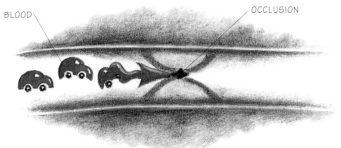

BLOOD

OCCLUSION

An artery that is completely blocked has no blood flowing through it. If the heart muscle does not receive blood, then it does not receive nutrients and oxygen. When the heart does

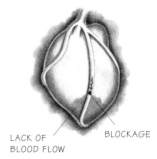

LACK OF
BLOOD FLOW

BLOCKAGE

not receive oxygen, it experiences **ischemia**. This may result in **heart pain** (angina) or a **heart attack. Ischemia**, if prolonged and severe enough, may cause a portion of the heart muscle to die.

What are some symptoms of a possible heart attack?

- **Angina**, or heart pain, usually felt as a pressure, ache, tightness, or **burning sensation** under the breastbone and often extending to the neck, jaw, shoulders, or down the arm (most frequently the left arm)
- **Nausea**
- **Shortness of breath** and/or **sweating**

Interestingly, **diabetic patients** do not "feel" angina in the same way and are more than twice as likely as nondiabetics to have a "silent" or unrecognized heart attack.

Quite often, people who are having a heart attack say they feel like "an elephant is standing on my chest."

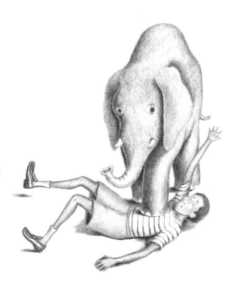

So, congestive heart failure may result when:

1) Coronary arteries become clogged.
2) Lack of blood causes a heart attack that damages the heart muscle (left ventricle), which then has a reduced pumping capacity.
3) An infection in the heart muscle (most frequently due to a virus) is unrecognized, and the heart muscle weakness or damage becomes evident at a later date.
4) High blood pressure is not properly controlled or an abnormal heart valve function (leaky or narrowed valve) exists.

What can be done to reduce your chances of developing heart disease?

Generally, cardiovascular disease takes a long time to develop. You may reduce your chances of developing heart disease by changing certain habits or "risk factors."

Risk Factors

The primary risk factors for cardiovascular disease include:

1) Elevated cholesterol

2) Smoking

3) Diabetes

4) Hypertension

5) Obesity

6) Family history

7) Age

8) Physical inactivity

1. Elevated cholesterol

Cholesterol is a "waxlike substance" that serves as a "building block" within the **cell membrane**.

CELL MEMBRANE

CHOLESTEROL

TESTOSTERONE

BILE ACID

ESTROGEN

Cholesterol is used to make **bile acids** that help break down fat in our intestines.

Cholesterol is also used to make **hormones,** especially those found in reproduction: **estrogen** and **testosterone**.

Why is cholesterol so harmful?

As mentioned, **fatty streaks** in the arteries start to develop in the first decade of life as a result of **lipids** moving into the cell wall of the artery. These fatty streaks may become more advanced **atherosclerotic lesions** and may then progress to "advanced lesions" often referred to as **plaque**.

Plaque restricts the flow of blood through the artery, similar to orange construction barrels you have seen on the highway. Plaque reduces the flow of blood (traffic) and increases pressure in the artery (construction zone).

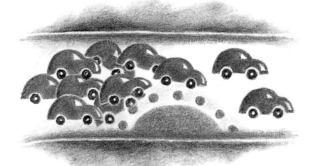

What should my cholesterol levels be?

For individuals who have coronary heart disease, the important number to remember is the **LDL-cholesterol**. For those individuals, **LDL-cholesterol** should be below **100 mg/dL**.

Triglycerides should be less than **200 mg/dL**.

HDL-cholesterol. For men, this value should be greater than **35 mg/dL**, and for women this value should be greater than **45 mg/dL**.

2. What about smoking?

Don't do it. Smoking is bad for the entire cardiovascular system because it:

A) Introduces carbon monoxide into the body

B) Lowers the "good" HDL-cholesterol

A. Carbon monoxide

Oxygen attaches to the red blood cells in the lungs. Red blood cells transport the oxygen throughout the body.

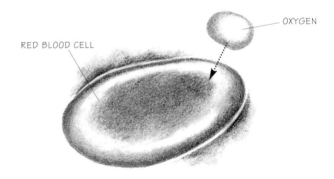

RED BLOOD CELL

OXYGEN

When you smoke, you inhale carbon monoxide into your lungs. Carbon monoxide binds to the red blood cells at the site where oxygen normally binds.

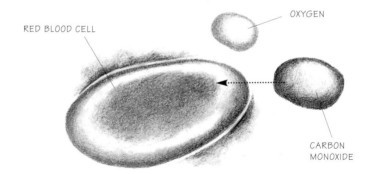

OXYGEN

RED BLOOD CELL

CARBON MONOXIDE

Therefore, less oxygen is carried by the blood, resulting in less oxygen available for use in the heart, muscles, and throughout the body. People who smoke may have abnormal heartbeats as well.

Understandably, smoking has harmful effects, especially for anyone who has already had a heart attack or bypass surgery. More importantly, there is an increased likelihood of a second heart attack or need for another bypass surgery if you continue to smoke after an initial cardiac incident.

B. Lower HDL-cholesterol

Two other reasons for not smoking are that it reduces the amount of HDL-cholesterol or "good cholesterol" in your bloodstream, and it makes your blood clot more easily, increasing the potential for an arterial blockage (heart attack or stroke).

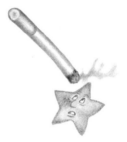

SMOKING
REDUCES
HDL-CHOLESTEROL

3. Diabetes

What exactly is diabetes? The working cells need sugar for energy. Sugar is absorbed through the digestive system after a meal or snack. **Insulin** is released by the **pancreas** to allow the body to use sugar as a source of nutrition and energy. That may be hard to visualize. This may help ...

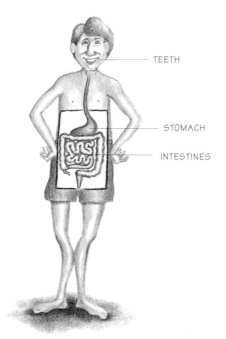

TEETH

STOMACH

INTESTINES

While you eat, the digestive system (teeth, stomach, and intestines) breaks your food down into smaller particles that are used by your body.

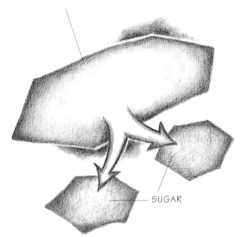

FOOD PARTICLE

SUGAR

Some food is broken down into particles of **sugar**. Sometimes this sugar is referred to as **carbohydrates** or **glucose**.

Sugar moves from the digestive system to the blood and travels throughout the body to feed the working cells. The sugar is the energy packet the cells need to do work like running and breathing.

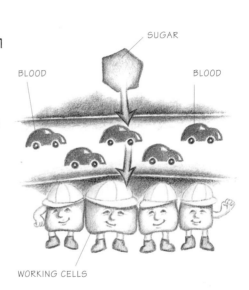

SUGAR

BLOOD

BLOOD

WORKING CELLS

At the same time, the body sends a signal to the **pancreas** telling it to release **insulin** into the bloodstream.

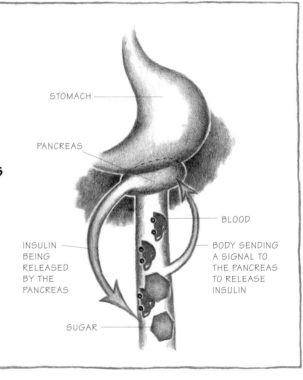

STOMACH

PANCREAS

BLOOD

INSULIN BEING RELEASED BY THE PANCREAS

BODY SENDING A SIGNAL TO THE PANCREAS TO RELEASE INSULIN

SUGAR

Insulin acts like a **key** that unlocks the doors of the cells to let sugar move in. The working cells can then use the sugar for energy to do their jobs. This is how your body uses sugar. However ...

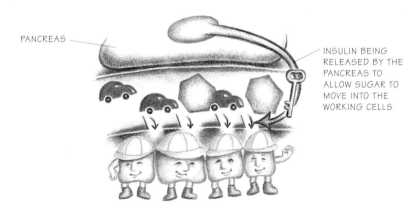

PANCREAS

INSULIN BEING RELEASED BY THE PANCREAS TO ALLOW SUGAR TO MOVE INTO THE WORKING CELLS

Without the key (insulin), the sugar cannot get out of the bloodstream and into the working cells. The sugar builds up in the blood, and the working cells get hungry. This is what happens in diabetes. A diabetic's body cannot move sugar from the blood into the cells.

Diabetes is a major risk factor for cardiovascular disease. Approximately 80% of diabetic patients eventually die of cardiovascular disease. It has been estimated that 50% of diabetics have some form of coronary heart disease prior to being diagnosed with diabetes.

4. Hypertension

SYSTOLIC NUMBER

140

90

DIASTOLIC NUMBER

Hypertension is commonly referred to as high blood pressure. If you have a **systolic pressure** greater than 140 mm Hg and/or a **diastolic pressure** greater than 90 mm Hg on 2 separate visits to the doctor, then you may have high blood pressure.

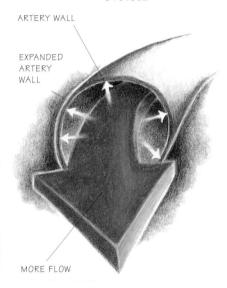

SYSTOLE

ARTERY WALL

EXPANDED ARTERY WALL

MORE FLOW

What is **systolic pressure**? Blood comes out of the heart in 1 big thrust. The artery expands to handle the blood. The amount of pressure put on the expanded artery wall is called **systolic pressure**.

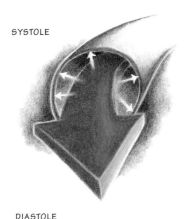

SYSTOLE

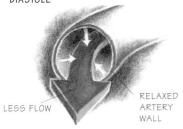

DIASTOLE

LESS FLOW

RELAXED ARTERY WALL

After the artery expands during systole, it relaxes back to its normal size. It is similar to a rubber band that goes back to its normal shape after being stretched. Normal pressure on the artery wall during relaxation is called **diastolic pressure**.

How *does* hypertension relate to cardiovascular disease?

Blood pressure is a result of the blood flowing through the artery (cardiac output) and the resistance of the artery wall (vascular resistance). If that sounds too technical, here ... this may help:

Blood pressure = Cardiac output x vascular resistance

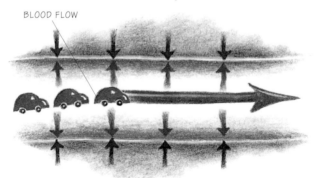

BLOOD FLOW

If a lot of resistance is created by either the blood or the artery wall, then there is more pressure as the blood travels through the artery. If it takes more energy to get the blood through the arteries, then your heart has to work harder with each beat. Most people with high blood pressure do not realize they have it. No wonder hypertension is called the "silent killer."

What contributes to hypertension?

Several factors may contribute to hypertension and cardiovascular disease. These include:

Excess dietary salt

Excess alcohol intake

Stress

Age

Genetics and family history

Obesity

Physical inactivity

High saturated fat diet

67

Salt

Salt helps conserve water in your body. The American Heart Association Step II Diet recommends that the average person consume no more than 2,400 mg of salt per day, especially those individuals who are salt sensitive. Excess dietary salt may contribute to both hypertension and to your body retaining too much water.

If you are retaining too much water, then you are increasing your blood volume (cars) without adding space. This increase will result in more pressure in the arteries.

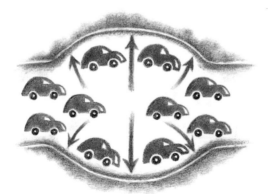

Alcohol consumption

A common concern for individuals with cardiovascular disease is alcohol consumption — mainly because there seems to be conflicting evidence about the benefits versus the risks of drinking. Experts agree that excess alcohol consumption over time can lead to many harmful effects, including high blood pressure, cirrhosis of the liver, and damage to the heart. The issue is the balance between **moderate** and **excessive** alcohol consumption.

While the evidence shows that there is a protective effect for moderate alcohol consumption, this benefit disappears with excessive intake. Men should consume no more than 2 drinks* daily, and women, because of their smaller body size, should not consume more than 1 drink* each day. The 7 to 14 allowable drinks in a week should not be consumed in a few days or during a weekend of binge drinking.

*A guide: One drink is defined as 5 ounces of wine, 12 ounces of beer, or 1-1/2 ounces of 80-proof liquor.

People who should not drink include individuals with high levels of triglycerides in their blood (over 300 mg/dL), women who are pregnant, individuals who are under age, people with a genetic predisposition for alcoholism or who are recovering from alcoholism, and those taking certain medications.

What about stress?

When you are under stress, your brain releases signals to the body through the nerves. These signals allow your body to respond to various situations.

Arteries have nerves attached to them. The nerves can either cause the arteries to relax or can put more tension on the walls of the arteries. If you are under a lot of stress, the nerves send signals to tighten or narrow the arteries.

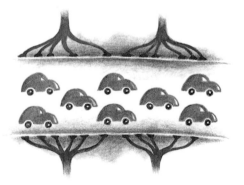

Narrowing the artery is like taking away a lane of traffic. There is still the same number of cars (blood) with less space (artery). This increases the pressure inside the artery.

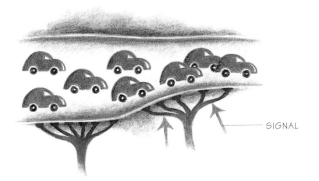

SIGNAL

So,

something you can do to improve your blood pressure is reduce stress. You can accomplish this by practicing meditation, doing deep breathing exercises, or doing exercise, such as going for a walk, riding a bike, or taking a swim.

5. Obesity

The American Heart Association has described obesity as a major risk factor for cardiovascular disease. What exactly is obesity?

Metropolitan Life's height/weight tables are often used to determine a recommended weight for an individual based on age and gender. Generally, those who are 20% over the recommended weight for their height are considered to be overweight — but not necessarily obese. Obesity refers to fatness rather than weight. Men who have greater than 25% of their body weight as fat and women who have more than 35% are considered to be obese. Obesity and being overweight carry significant health risks, are directly related to cardiovascular risk factors, and may:

1) raise triglycerides (a "bad" blood fat)
2) lower HDL-cholesterol (the "good" cholesterol)
3) raise LDL-cholesterol (the "bad" cholesterol)
4) raise blood pressure and
5) increase the risk of developing diabetes

Obesity may be related to both genetics (nature) and lifestyle (nurture). Generally speaking, obesity occurs when the calories we consume exceed the calories we burn through activities of daily living and exercise. We store the excess calories as fat reserves, thus contributing to obesity and ultimately increasing the risk of coronary disease. Obesity has increased in men and women in every decade over the past 50 years.

There is a misconception that Americans are overeating and eating too much fat. In fact, as a nation we are eating less fat, fewer calories, and still gaining weight — primarily due to the lower levels of physical activity in our youth and adult lives. A sedentary life could be the real culprit.

6. Family history

A **family history** of cardiovascular disease could reflect genetics and/or an unhealthy family lifestyle. If most of your family members smoke, are sedentary, and have a poor diet — then these are harmful habits that increase the risk of heart disease in your family. However, unlike your genes, these behaviors can be changed.

On the other hand, if your family has a healthful lifestyle but there is still a high incidence of cardiovascular disease, then it is likely that genetics is playing a role. In either case, by practicing a healthful lifestyle, you can help reduce your risk rather than giving up and thinking you have no control over your destiny.

7. Age

Aging has an effect on the risk of cardiovascular disease because aging causes changes in the heart and blood vessels. As people age, they become less active, gain more weight, and the effects of a sedentary lifestyle, smoking, and poor diet continue to damage the heart and circulation by increasing blood pressure and cholesterol levels. Blood pressure increases with aging, in part because arteries gradually lose some of their elasticity and, over time, may not be as resilient.

8. Physical inactivity

Lack of exercise is a major contributor to obesity, diabetes, and hypertension. Beginning an exercise program may help you feel better, help you have more energy, help you lose some weight, lower your cholesterol, lower your blood pressure, help you look better, and improve your muscle tone. Also, beginning an exercise routine can increase your HDL-cholesterol or "good cholesterol" — especially if exercise is associated with weight loss.

Exercise

Our discussion will be separated into 2 parts:

- Exercise for those who have CHF and

- Exercise for those who do not have CHF but who may be at risk of developing CHF

For those who have CHF

1) You should be evaluated by your doctor. Usually a doctor will use a stress test to determine your exercise limitations.

2) After the stress test, your cardiologist should be able to recommend an appropriate exercise intensity for your exercise program. If you have not exercised in a long time, start off very slowly. You may want to try walking or stationary cycling. A good way to begin is with **intervals**. What is **interval training**? Keep reading. Always follow your doctor's advice regarding exercise.

Interval training example

Week 1

Each exercise session should consist of walking or cycling for 1 minute and recovering by walking slowly or cycling slowly for 1 minute. Repeat this between 5 and 10 times. Try to exercise for a total of 10 to 15 minutes each day.

Week 2

Walk or cycle 1-1/2 minutes and rest 1 minute. Again, repeat this between 5 and 10 times each day. Adding one-half minute to each interval length will gradually increase your exercise capacity.

How hard and how often should I exercise?

When you are just starting out, try to exercise very comfortably. Here are 4 quick tips.

1) Try to exercise so that you are breathing noticeably but are **not** out of breath. Remember this simple rule: you should be able to carry on a conversation while you are exercising.

2) Sweating is a good thing. This means that your body is working hard enough and receiving the necessary stimulus for the muscles and the heart.

3) If you are not fatigued and are completely recovered from exercising on the previous day, then you should exercise **daily**.

4) Give yourself a **warm-up** before exercise (several minutes of easy walking) and a **cooldown** at the end of exercise (again, several minutes of easy walking). Ask an exercise specialist for some recommendations for stretching after your workout, and discuss the intensity of the exercise with your doctor. **If you feel any chest discomfort, discontinue your exercise and consult your doctor.**

What if I **do not** have CHF?

Actually, a lot of the same principles apply.

1) Ask your doctor for a stress test prior to beginning an exercise routine. Before beginning, discuss the nature and type of exercise routine with your doctor.

2) Begin with a simple interval training program. You may gradually increase the time by 1 minute each week.

Sample interval training schedule

Week 1   1 minute walking or cycling/
1 minute rest for 5 to 10 intervals

Week 2   2 minutes walking or cycling/
1 minute rest for 5 to 10 intervals

Week 3   3 minutes walking or cycling/
1 minute rest for 5 to 10 intervals

A reasonable goal would be to gradually increase
your exercise routine over 6 weeks until you are
exercising 20 to 30 minutes comfortably each day.

Again, remember:

1) Be sure to give yourself at least 5 minutes of easy warm-up and cooldown. You may also want to add some light stretching exercises.

2) **Discontinue exercising if you feel chest discomfort, and consult your doctor.**

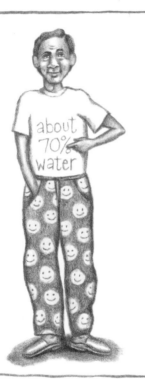

Another consideration — water

Water is needed for virtually every function of the body. The body is approximately 70% water.

With congestive heart failure, retaining additional water may make your condition worse. Your doctor may ask you to limit your intake of fluid to no more than 48 ounces per day.

Check with your doctor to see what your fluid limitations should be.

Medications,
Angioplasty,
and
Bypass Surgery

What if changing your risk factors and beginning an exercise program do not help?

What's next?

Your doctor may refer you to a heart specialist called a **cardiologist**. The cardiologist may have to consider several options including **medications** or surgical intervention such as **angioplasty** or **bypass surgery**.

Some commonly
prescribed classifications
of medications used with
congestive heart failure

Digitalis

When the heart beats, it contracts forcefully to pump out the blood. If the heart has been damaged, the force of the contraction may have been reduced. Digitalis (or digoxin) acts to increase the force with which the left ventricle contracts.

Diuretics

Blood is 92% water. If the kidneys cannot properly remove excess water, the blood volume will be increased. This results in fluid retention with subsequent shortness of breath and edema. Diuretics target the kidneys. They help to eliminate excess water and decrease the overall blood volume as well as reduce shortness of breath and edema.

ACE (angiotensin converting enzyme) inhibitors, All (angiotensin receptor) blockers and vasodilators

Say that 3 times fast! These drugs act to enlarge the diameter of the arteries (reduce vascular resistance), thereby permitting an easier flow of blood and decreasing the workload of the heart. These drugs may vary with respect to their peak effective daily dose and the required frequency of administration.

Beta blockers

When the heart fails, the body increases levels of **adrenaline** in the blood in an attempt to stimulate the heart muscle to work harder. Over time, adrenaline fatigues the heart and has a negative effect. Beta blockers can "block" the effect of adrenaline on the heart muscle and may prevent heart muscle deterioration. Beta-blocker therapy should be started at low doses and must be carefully monitored by your doctor.

Cholesterol-lowering and antiplatelet therapy

If congestive heart failure is due to a heart attack and coronary artery disease, medications typically prescribed to treat coronary artery disease (cholesterol-lowering medicines and aspirin) may reduce the likelihood of recurrent cardiac events (ischemia and heart attack).

Angioplasty

Angioplasty may provide benefits to patients with CHF
if a significant degree of heart muscle dysfunction is
due to ischemia, which can be relieved when angioplasty
opens the coronary blockage. Angioplasty is a procedure
by which the cardiologist inserts a balloon catheter over
a thin wire across a blockage of a coronary artery.

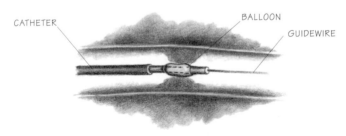

CATHETER   BALLOON   GUIDEWIRE

The balloon is inflated to compress the plaque. This is repeated as necessary by the cardiologist.

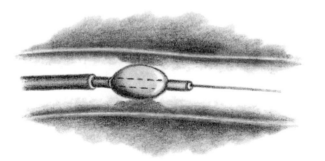

Inflating the catheter compresses and breaks apart the plaque. This allows more room for the blood to flow.

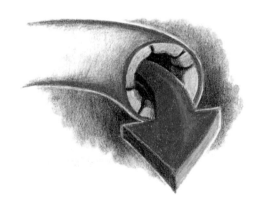

The balloon catheter also stretches the elastic wall of the artery. Small tears occur on the inside of the artery wall and slightly injure the artery wall as a result of balloon catheter inflation.

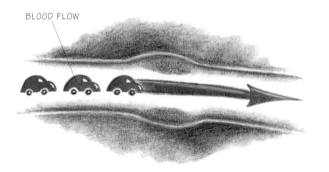

BLOOD FLOW

Unfortunately, these balloon catheter injuries expose substances from inside the atherosclerotic plaque and the artery wall that promote formation of blood clots.

Complications of this procedure may include a heart attack, repeat angioplasty, the need for emergency coronary bypass surgery, and even death.

Stents

In certain instances, the cardiologist may decide to insert a **stent** inside the coronary artery. The stent, usually made of stainless steel, functions as a scaffold to hold open the inside of the coronary artery.

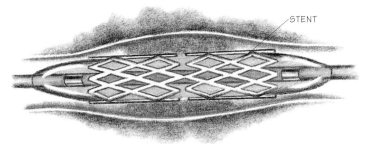

STENT

Stents are usually put in place using a balloon angioplasty catheter. Stents can reduce the incidence of both short- and long-term coronary artery reocclusion. Stents can seal and "tack up" tissue flaps within the artery that are created when a balloon catheter injures the artery. Unfortunately, stents do not eliminate clot formation or the occurrence of heart attack following the procedure.

Valve replacement

The valves inside the heart are one-way valves. For instance, the mitral valve allows blood to flow from the left atrium into the left ventricle.

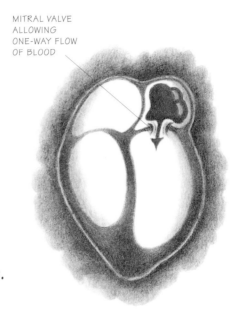

MITRAL VALVE ALLOWING ONE-WAY FLOW OF BLOOD

When the left ventricle contracts, the mitral valve closes and the blood travels out to the body through the aorta.

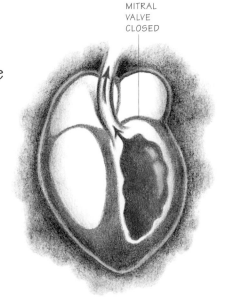

MITRAL
VALVE
CLOSED

If the mitral valve loses some of its integrity or ability to close properly, then the blood may flow back into the left atrium when the left ventricle contracts. This leakage of the valve is called **mitral regurgitation**.

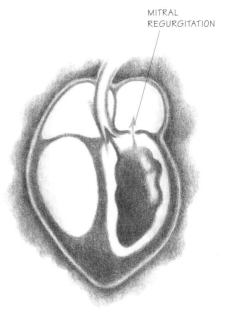

MITRAL REGURGITATION

If mitral regurgitation occurs over a prolonged period of time, the left ventricle works harder and harder to pump blood forward to the body and, with time, muscle damage occurs. A similar situation may involve the aortic valve as well. Heart valve failure may contribute to congestive heart failure.

Are there any surgical options to repair the valve? A cardiac surgeon may repair either valve or, in certain instances, cut out the old valve and replace it with a new one. Repairing the valve may help prevent the blood from flowing back into the left atrium and can restore more normal (one-way) valve function.

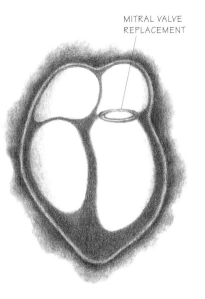

MITRAL VALVE REPLACEMENT

Bypass surgery

Bypass surgery is a cardiovascular procedure designed to correct blood flow to the heart that angioplasty cannot correct. The cardiovascular surgeon uses a piece of artery and/or vein to reroute blood around the blockage. Patients with CHF may benefit from bypass surgery if reversible ischemia is the cause of heart muscle dysfunction.

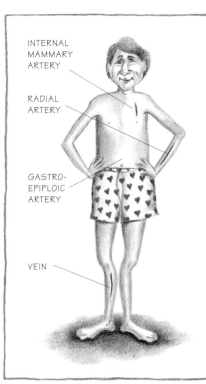

INTERNAL
MAMMARY
ARTERY

RADIAL
ARTERY

GASTRO-
EPIPLOIC
ARTERY

VEIN

The surgeon may use a vein from the leg, and/or the internal mammary artery found in the chest, and/or the gastroepiploic artery of the stomach, and/or the radial artery of the forearm.

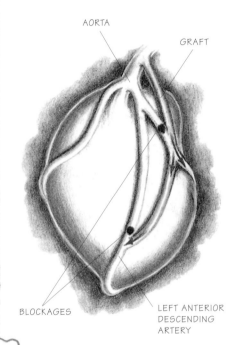

AORTA

GRAFT

BLOCKAGES

LEFT ANTERIOR
DESCENDING
ARTERY

The vein is attached to the aorta. The supply of blood is then rerouted around the blockage. One piece of vein may be used for multiple bypasses. The number of blockages where blood has been rerouted — not the number of veins used — determines the number of bypasses.

If the internal mammary artery is used, the artery originates from a branch off the aorta and is attached directly below the blockage.

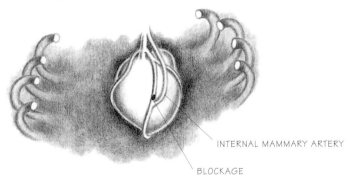

INTERNAL MAMMARY ARTERY

BLOCKAGE

Heart transplant

What happens if the left ventricle has been severely damaged by a heart attack or infection? Is there anything else that can be done?

In certain instances, an individual's only hope of survival may be to receive a heart transplant. There are many critical issues that determine who is a candidate for a transplant.

Despite advances in technology, no cardiac procedure is without some inherent risk for the patient. These may include, but are not limited to:

- heart attack
- stroke
- infection
- bleeding or hemorrhaging
- abnormal heart rhythm
- death

What about 'after care' from a heart attack, bypass surgery, or angioplasty?

Your doctor will manage your care very closely. Generally, the cardiologist may recommend that you:

- quit smoking
- take a beta blocker drug (after a heart attack)
- lower your LDL-cholesterol below 100 mg/dL
- take a daily enteric-coated aspirin (81 mg or greater) unless you have other medical complications
- follow a "heart-healthy diet" and begin a basic exercise program, mainly walking. Always follow your doctor's recommendations.

Questions

Here are some questions that you may want to take with you the next time you go to see your doctor.

What are my medications? How does each of them help me?

Answer _____

_____

_____

_____

_____

_____

_____

_____

List the blood pressure reading for each visit to your doctor and the date.

Date	Blood Pressure
_____	_____
_____	_____
_____	_____
_____	_____
_____	_____
_____	_____

Do I have any *exercise limitations* of which I should be aware? What are they?

Answer _____

_____

Should I have a *treadmill test* before I start to exercise? What is my target heart rate?

Answer _____

_____

Based on my weight, blood pressure, and blood cholesterol level, should I talk to someone about changing my diet?

Yes   No

Contact your local hospital for the name of a registered dietitian.

Dietitian _____

Address _____

_____

Phone _____

Are there any concerns that I should be aware of before having/resuming sexual activity?

Answer

_____

_____

_____

_____

And now for a little heart to heart ...

There are any number of reasons why someone may develop congestive heart failure. They range from a heart attack to contracting an infection of the heart muscle to high blood pressure.

The point is this. If you have had a cardiac event, or if you think you may be at risk for cardiovascular disease, **now** is the time to take command of your life. We cannot control the past, but we can control what we do today and beyond.

Go see your doctor and have a complete physical exam. If necessary, sit down with a dietitian and review your current eating patterns. Then, if your doctor agrees, get moving. Start a simple exercise program — mainly walking. There are no guarantees that you will reduce your risk of having a cardiac event, but at least you will be taking an aggressive approach to improving your health.

Bibliography

American College of Sports Medicine position stand. "The Recommended Quality and Quantity of Exercise for Developing and Maintaining Cardiorespiratory and Muscular Fitness in Healthy Adults." *Medicine and Science in Sports and Exercise* April 1990.

American Heart Association Consensus Panel Statement. "Preventing Heart Attack and Death in Patients With Coronary Disease." *Circulation* 1995; 2-4.

Angell, M. "Caring for women's health – What is the problem?" *New England Journal of Medicine* 1993: 271.

Burke, A.P., and A. Farb, G.T. Malcom, Y. Liang, J. Smialek, R. Virmani. "Coronary Risk Factors and Plaque Morphology in Men with Coronary Disease Who Died Suddenly." *New England Journal of Medicine* 1 May 1997: 1276-1282.

Cogswell, M.E. "Nicotine Withdrawal Symptoms." *North Carolina Medical Journal* 1 Jan. 1995: 40-45.

Collins, R., and R. Peto, C. Baigent, P. Sleight. "Aspirin, Heparin, and Fibrinolytic Therapy in Suspected Acute Myocardial Infarction." *New England Journal of Medicine* 20 March 1997: 847-860.

Da Costa, F.D., et al. "Myocardial Revascularization with the Radial Artery: A Clinical and Angiographic Study." *Annals of Thoracic Surgery* Aug. 1996: 475-480.

Eckel, R.H. "Obesity in Heart Disease." *Circulation* 1997: 3248-3250.

Friedman, G.D., and A.L. Klatsky. "Is Alcohol Good for Your Health?" *New England Journal of Medicine* 16 Dec. 1993: 1882-1883.

Gellar, A. "Common Addictions." *Clinical Symposia.* Ciba-Geigy Corporation 1996.

Grossman, E., and F.H. Messerli. "Diabetic and Hypertensive Heart Disease." *Annals of Internal Medicine* 15 Aug. 1996: 304-310.

Henningfield, J.D., and R.M. Keenan. "The Anatomy of Nicotine Addiction." *Health Values* March/April 1993: 12-19.

Joint National Committee. The Fifth Report of the Joint National Committee on Detection, Evaluation, and Treatment of High Blood Pressure. Bethesda (MD): National Institutes of Health, National Heart, Lung, and Blood Institute; 1993. NIH publication No. 93-1008.

Kannel, W.B., and R.B. D'Agostino, J.L. Cobb. "Effects of Weight on Cardiovascular Disease." *American Journal of Clinical Nutrition* March 1996: 419S-422S.

Kenney, W.L. et al. *American College of Sports Medicine Guidelines for Exercise Testing and Prescription.* 5th ed. Media, Pa.: Williams & Wilkins, 1995.

Margolis, S., and P.J. Goldschmidt-Clermont. *The Johns-Hopkins White Papers.* Baltimore: The Johns-Hopkins Medical Institutions, 1996.

McCarron, D.A., and M.E. Reusser. "Body Weight and Blood Pressure Regulation." *American Journal of Clinical Nutrition* March 1996: 423S-425S.

Meeker, M.H., and J.C. Rothrock. *Alexander's Care of the Patient in Surgery,* 10th ed. St. Louis: Mosby, 1995.

Peterson, J.A., and C.X. Bryant, *The Fitness Handbook; 2nd edition,* St. Louis: Wellness Bookshelf, 1995.

Ryan, T.J., and J.L. Anderson, E.M. Autman, et al. "ACC/AHA Guidelines for the Management of Patients with Acute Myocardial Infarction: A Report of the American College of Cardiology/American Heart Association Task Force on Practice Guidelines (Committee on Management of Acute Myocardial Infarction)." *Journal of the American College of Cardiology* 1 Nov. 1996: 1328-1428.

St. Jeor, S.T., and K.D. Brownell, R.L. Atkinson, C. Bouchard, et al. "Obesity Workshop III." *Circulation* 1996: 1391-1396.

Schlant, R.C., and R.W. Alexander. *The Heart*, 8th ed. New York: McGraw-Hill, 1994.

Superko, H.R. "The Most Common Cause of Coronary Heart Disease can be Successfully Treated by the Least Expensive Therapy — Exercise." *Certified News* 1998: 1-5.

United States Surgeon General. Department of Health and Human Services. *The Health Consequences of Smoking. Nicotine Addiction.* Washington, D.C.: U.S. Department of Health and Human Services, 1988.

United States Surgeon General on his priorities at http://www.osophs.dhhs.gov/myjob/priorities.htm accessed November 1999.

Voors, A.A., et al. "Smoking and Cardiac Events After Venous Coronary Bypass Surgery." *Circulation* Jan 1, 1995: 42-47.

Voutilainen, S., et al. "Angiographic 5-Year Follow-up Study of Right Gastroepiploic Artery Grafts." *Annals of Thoracic Surgery* Aug. 1996: 501-505.

White H.D., and J.J. Van de Werf. "Thrombolysis for Acute Myocardial Infarction." *Circulation* 28 April 1998: 1632-1646.

Zelasko, C.J. "Exercise for Weight Loss: What are the Facts?" *Journal of the American Dietetic Association* Dec. 1995: 973-1031.

For additional copies of
Congestive Heart Failure: What You Should Know™,
contact your local bookseller
or call: (800) 289-0963.

For institutional quantities, call Joanne Widmer
at (800) 666-0963 ext. 262.
Other titles in the series *Your Health: What You Should Know*™:

Heart Disease: What You Should Know™
Diabetes: What You Should Know™
High Cholesterol: What You Should Know™
Women's Health Under 40: What You Should Know™
Women's Health Over 40: What You Should Know™